Table of Contents

Copyright

Safety & Infection Control

OB & Maternity

Pediatrics & Development

Psychosocial

Topics: Endocrine

Topics: Neurology

Topics: Renal

Topics: Hematology

Topics: Cardiology

Topics: Respiratory

Topics: Musculoskeletal & Integumentary

Topics: Gastrointestinal

Topics: Oncology

Labs & Interpretation

Pharmacology

Author's Note

If you're reading this, you've come a long way. Many hours studying… Many hours learning and gaining important experience. It is now time to take the most formidable test of them all: the NCLEX-RN. You're worried. On test day: how many questions will you get? Will I run out of time? Should I take breaks?… Will I pass?

We are all to familiar with his roller-coaster of emotions. This exam is daunting even for the best students. But after hours of studying... And 75 to 145 computer adaptive questions messing with your head... You will know the answer to the almighty question.

Whether your exam is a year away or literally tomorrow, we at Cambridge 10 have been there with you all. Most of us are pre-meds, nurses and doctors who are passionate about helping care for and being of service to real people. Many of us faced the same challenge you did to get there. The long hours studying, the stress, and the quintessential NCLEX. Either way, we understand one fundamental fact. It is an illusion that anyone who takes this well prepared. Whether you studied for 1 weeks or 1 years in advance, everyone gets hit with some curve-balls no matter how many practice questions, flashcards, or expensive courses you've taken.

What we realized after every hopeless 10+ hour study day and all the exam room anxiety is the following. No one needs yet another test prep book with 700 reworded practice questions. No one needs tips like "eat a granola bar!", "make sure to bring water!" In short, no one needs something the regurgitated study tips, or 20-year-old notes, or another time-sink that only makes your studies more difficult and confusing. If your serious about this test, you have enough of those challenges already. Instead, we realized that we needed, in addition to the practice test, question banks, and so on... Something that shortcuts the long path to learning...That builds new connections that save us time and energy but still keep us focused. And lastly, that allows some creativity and positivity amidst the sleepless, draining study nights.

Thus, this book is about solving one problem and one problem only: how to keep that god-almighty massive amount of information in our tiny little brains to win at this exam. No deep critical thinking here, just quick memory shortcuts that allow our prefrontal cortex to live to fight another day. *This* is the key. A small shortcut, a small optimization that adds up, saving in the end lots of time and mental energy. This is simple breakthrough we figured out after we testing dozens of ideas. After refining a study and memory strategy and developing on aspiring nurses of all backgrounds, we had a blueprint to get little knowledge and preparation to pass the NCLEX *and* keep the real knowledge that helps you succeed as an RN.

Let us be clear, the path we take in this book is *not* a silver bullet that effortlessly gets you that magic number you envision on your score report. The process we outline requires intentionality, creativity, and awareness even... No *especially* on study days you feel most exhausted. We can't offer magic, but we can offer a foundation that has been battle-tested by many, us included, that you can build on through discipline and creativity to accelerate your score improvement.

On the flip side, our key strategy of remembering and personalizing your own mnemonics can be fun and creative aspect of your studies... A break from the drudgery of critically thinking to anxiously converge on an answer on your 700th practice question. In fact, the best mnemonics are like little mind viruses. They are created by you and only to benefit you. They can be right there when you need them many years later when you've secured your dream, and want nothing to do with the NCLEX ever again.

So, we hope to have convinced you a little on how underrated mnemonics really are. This is *the* important belief you need going into the NCLEX. It allows you to buy into storing mnemonics in a brain that initially wants to forget it. This belief allows you to creatively generate mnemonics, to visualize them, to create a story for them, to place them in your unique mind. The specific testing-backed strategies and research-supported processes for implementing these memory tricks in your study we will discuss in the next section **How to Use**.

Overall, this is a deceptively simple book... An index of some good mnemonics. But, it is up to you to adopt our tried-and-tested study process. You will need to fill in the blanks. You need to buy into creating a memory system that saves mental effort for the questions/sections that matter most... To literally have fun remembering things *and* succeed at using them. For this reason we provide specific strategies and outline a study process that incorporates this book with others resources to maximizes your success. The mental tricks in this book, and those that you write on your own, should offset the pain of having a random encyclopedia of lab values jumbling around in your head. We hope you can use these tools to succeed. We hope to encourage the part of you that says, *"I can do this."*

We hope you enjoy this book. If you found it at all useful please leave us a ★★★★★ wherever you found us. If you have any feedback on how to improve, email us at support@cambridgeten.com. We are a small startup team of students and professionals with a mission **to give ambitious people real strategies to help them succeed on any exam**.

If you are interested in a complete NCLEX-RN study platform, **sign up and create a study plan at cambridgeten.com.** The coupon below gets you 20% off a monthly subscription! If you notice errors in the book, email us, and whenever we update it we will send you a free updated e-book copy and refund your test prep subscription. Thanks for reading. We're rooting for you!

Sincerely,

The Cambridge Ten Team

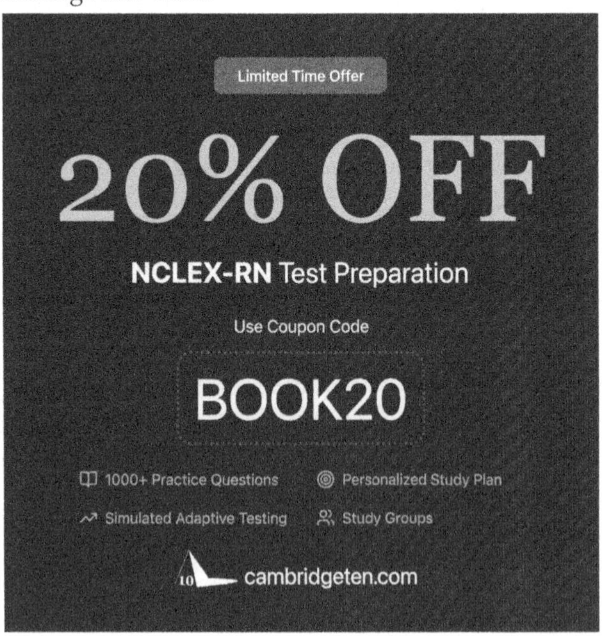

How to Use

What is this book?

This book is an index of the most popular an effective mnemonics for the NCLEX exam. It is split up into sections representing each medical topic on the exam, not necessarily the exam sections. Based on our insights with students, we found that mirroring the way they naturally studied was far more broken-down and memorable than the sections of the NCLEX, which are simply too broad. However, it is worth looking at their categories to understand the underlying philosophy of the exam. We go into this later.

The reason for this setup is also to help you use this as a resource after you have completed the NCLEX. A simple reference guide to pick up and get to where you need to go. Overall, this book is meant to be flipped through as you study and do practice questions so you can easily search for something you need, and later as a simplified reference

The Blank Pages, Make Your Own

The blank pages at the end of each section are meant for you to fill in, add your own mnemonics, write down group-study notes, etc. They should be related to the mnemonic on the right, even if only tangentially. Let's run through some examples:

- *"The mnemonic for this sucks! I have my own!"*: This is great! Feel free to get a giant marker and scribble out our entire page and write your mnemonic down on the blank page. In fact, we find many do this for vulgar mnemonics, which can be sharper triggers of memory (... if that's your thing of course)

- *"I want to write a little cheat sheet for questions/topics related to this mnemonic"*: This is useful, but understand that simplicity is key. Cramming all the information onto a single page like you do for school exams won't work well. Our strategy is to create more shortcuts for your brain to remember as opposed to spending excess mental energy. For this reason, we recommend making sure the content is a mnemonic, rhyme, ordered list, drawing, etc. Anything that has a well defined pattern, emotional connection, visualization, or all of those at the same time.

- *"I don't care about your system, I'll write whatever I want!"*: Thats totally OK. After all, these are just guide lines, not a double-blind randomized controlled trials. No matter what you want to do, remember to be aware if it is working for you, otherwise cut it. For example, we found that students that created a **5 Principle Study Plan** (the next section) were more committed and more positive throughout the study and test-taking process. So... if you end up not using this book, thats alright! As long as you take-away that the path to success is you putting that systematic effort in even under stress and constraint. That is what we believe will train you to stay diligent and positive on the long road to NCLEX and actual nursing success.

So, I hope you understand the importance of these blank pages. Remember that it doesn't have to be perfect. In fact, most students we tested wrote on less than half of the blank pages. However, those that wrote at least 1 or 2 small things on at least 30% of the blank pages tended to perform significantly better than the others. As you take on your study, primarily when you are doing content review, take advantage of developing your internal bank of mnemonics early and often. The more questions on which you recall the mnemonic, even when not related to the answering the question, allows it to transfer into long-term memory.

The Study Plan

Now that we have understood how to use this book and even populate it with our own memory tricks, let's look at testing strategy. These are strategies we have tested extensively by running NCLEX tutoring and content review programs for students of all backgrounds.

First, once you have selected your test-date, reverse engineer your schedule. What time commitments do you have? School? Work? Personal time? You need 200 hours of studying *minimum*, so do the math and see how many hours each day or week you can commit given your respective time commitments. Your goal should be able to do a minimum of 50 questions every day. The goal is consistency as opposed to overloading on questions on any given day. So, it is ideal to find a consistent time block that you can commit to every day... If you can. If the math isn't adding up, you will unfortunately need to make a sacrifice in other activities, even if it is for more personal time to rest and rejuvenate. Remember that studying should push you out of your comfort zone, and that it is ultimately temporary.

Study Resources

Study resources are an instrumental aspect of success on the NCLEX, but no particular study resource trumps out all the rest. The key resource types are: question banks, content review programs and personal memory tools.

Question banks are the bedrock of your studying, so you should ideally have at least two recently-updated question banks from whatever test-prep companies. Choose one your friend has, or do whatever research you need to figure out which one you want. Completely up to you.

However, it is content review programs where you should do more research into what you might like. Some like the structure of paid test prep sites, whereas some find success in specific free YouTube teachers. Since we don't know you, you have to reflect on your learning style yourself, and what additional resources you might need (tutoring, group review sessions, disabilities, etc).

The third and final resource, personal memory tools, is where we come in. This resource represents all the tools you use to retain knowledge effectively. Again, everyone is different, some like online flashcards, others can survive simply on a notebook and a pencil. However, we believe this book can serve as a vital instrument to your NCLEX study journey. In particular, the specificity of the memory tricks we provide, as well as the ones you make yourself, will give you an easy reference as you tackle the frequent unknown concept or context in a NCLEX case. In the end, you will have a strong base of shortcuts to apply on test day and beyond to safely operate as a Registered Nurse. Now that we have established the relevant resources, let's get to tactical studying strategies you can apply on your study schedule you committed to.

Day 1 (Practice Test 1)

It's your day one, your first day. If you are excited and ready to get into it, congratulations, this will be your easiest day of all. If you begin to sit down and feel immense dread on opening your computer or prep or book, congratulations, this will be your hardest day of all. For the dreaders, we recommend that you take a few minutes to write... speculate about why you might feel that way. It seems trivial, but it tends to help you work through those feelings over the next days. Now that you have an idea of the psychological tools, lets get to tactical strategies.

The key way we have achieved success for NCLEX exam takers is to replicate the exam environment at least 3 times throughout your study journey. Thus, your first day will involve taking the full test, at the "worst" case scenario: 150 questions in 5 hours. Operating with this "worst" case is critically important because it allows you to conquer a central anxiety of test-takers. "How many questions until the computer tells me i'm done?" Then, if you have only done a couple questions a day to practice, the stress eats away at you. After question 75, you begin to ruminate, and it only gets stronger as you continue and get more fatigued. This undoubtedly affects your ability to answer questions effectively. At worst, your lack of comfort causes you to speed through questions on purpose! Because this is an adaptive exam, you must avoid this mistake at all costs, as this is the worst possible one. For this reason, re-frame your expectations. You will be answering 150 questions in 5 hours. Any earlier finish is a nice bonus. And for this reason, we expect you to stick by replicating a practice test environment where you answer, well, 150 questions in 5 hours. Please stick by this, even if you are tired, it's late, or any excuse you may have. It will make you sharper!

Now, as to what questions or resources to use for your first practice exam, this will be highly dependent on your resources. Think like your designing an experiment. How would you pick the questions? Would you pick questions of this specific topic only? or multiple? Would you pick only multiple choice questions or ones with a variety of answer types? (drag and drop, fill in the blank, etc.) Hopefully, you recognize the necessity of choosing a diversity of questions in multiple topic areas. Because of the diversity, you will be able to be confident in your improvement as you take further practice tests. So, there are a variety of ways to tackle this based on your resources. If you get an online NCLEX question bank, which we recommend, get ones with a feature where you can form a practice quiz/exam of 150 random questions of any type/topic/difficulty. Another alternative that can be more specific are online NCLEX diagnostic exams, whereby they can highlight specific topics you struggle in. Make sure you can't see whether your question is right or wrong until the very end, and that your not reusing questions you have already seen (usually online platforms have features to turn this off.)

Ensure when you take your first 150 questions that you develop a very exam-like environment. Clear your desk. Turn your phone off and put it away the entire session (hard I know). Only allow taking breaks once you are 2 hours into the exam, and do not pause the timer for any reason. Have snacks, food, and drink pre-prepared if you want to consume them on your break. And seriously, no phone!

Once you are done with 150 long, hard, painful questions, you are done for the day! Take the fattest break or self-care night, whatever you feel is rewarding you for a hard first day's work.

Day 2 (Reviewing Practice Test 1)

It is day 2. Hopefully you took a well-deserved break. Now you have to go through each question of your practice test one by one. Go through each question and note the question type and topic. If you took an online exam or a diagnostic one specifically, this should be easier. Of course, also as you go through each question, focus on why you got questions right as well as why you got questions wrong. If there are explanations, great. If not, take more time to see if you can walk through the logic that gets you to the correct answer. Write all aspects of this post-exam reflection down in your notes. In particular, when you are done going through the questions, note the most common question types and topics that you got something's wrong, as well as any other reflections you have on the exam. This is critical so you can design a real review plan that addresses your personally challenging topics. You should be spending at least an hour for this whole process, even if you may feel disappointed in your exam performance. The process of improvement is all that there is in this NCLEX marathon

! So put your ego of a low score away. Instead, set a baseline so that your score, no matter how low, gives you faith you will only go onward and upward! The score isn't the brag. The change in score (and your confidence) is, and you are building the foundation right now.

High Content Phase:

Now it's time to dive into the content. This phase is the first half of your study plan duration. Here you need to focus 80% on content and 20% on practice (in the next phase, these will flip). We recommend using online content review resources that extensively separate by content. If you do this, keep a notepad/notebook beside you as you go through online content. This will keep you in the habit of annotating, writing mnemonics, and other tactile methods to engage memory and actually use the whiteboard during the exam to recover memory and externalize your logic. However, using books for this is still very effective, and can help if you feel like studying on a screen makes you distractable.

Regardless of either option, we recommend creating an Excel table or some other type of organized note of all chapters the book(s) you have procured to use covering all NCLEX content. The goal is to help you easily move around organize topics based on your reflections on Practice Test 1, and prevent you from just going linearly through the book or online content review course, which would be very inefficient and not personal to your needs.

Based on our exam preparation programs, here are more strategies to consider:

- Go through each subject of content review in the order organized by your reflection from Practice Test 1. Then, reverse the order. This ensures you have the most challenging topic on the topic of your mind when you take the next practice test. If this doesn't work with your study schedule, condense 2 -3 topics into a study day, particularly if you feel very strongly about these topics.

- If you can stomach the long hours, try to review your practice test immediately or the same day of your practice test. This will shorten the feedback of you connecting your thinking on that question to the correct logic, making you improve faster. However if you can't pay attention or are too fatigued, stop and do it the next day. A weekend can often be a good time for this since you can spend time with friends or do other things later in the day to relax with relatively less stress from other commitments hanging over you.

- If feeling overwhelmed or frustrated by the difficult of the content, alternate between easy and hard days. That is, modify your study plan so that tomorrow you are doing content review subject you feel confident in. Alternatively, if you did 40 questions today in one subject, do 20 questions tomorrow on the next subject. This is a marathon, and giving yourself a small break can help you not burn out, as long as you commit to going back to the original study pace that makes you feel a little uncomfortable.

- Be diligent about the work. This exam rewards breadth of applicable knowledge... So you need to apply all the knowledge available. This is the make-or-break phase where good study skills and time-management form and shine. Your best improvements will likely come from this period. You will be enticed to add push off today's work tomorrow, but this is a cartoonishly slippery slope that we've seen many fall behind on. If you need to update your plan, update early and be honest with yourself. Commit to the dates, and reward yourself at the end of the day or on an off-day for sticking to the program.

Practice Test 2-3: Depending on your schedule, your next practice tests should be taken midway through or at the end of the High Content Phase. Whichever is more convenient. Ideally, take only one test at the end. If your schedule is longer, say longer than a month, then take one at the end and take another at the midpoint of the High Practice Phase described after this. The test or tests are extremely important as they complete the feedback loop. They highlight what content you focus on thereafter, and the depth of knowledge you may honestly be lacking in specific topics. After taking a practice test, take the next day off again as a reward.

High Practice Phase:

This will be the latter half of your study plan duration: 80% practice 20% content. At this point you will mostly be taking practice exams/ sections and reviewing content you missed (for example question topics that you missed in earlier practice exams). Remember: every step of the feedback loop is important. You will be tempted to breeze through whether you got the answers right or wrong, when in fact you should be deep diving on each question, particularly ones you got wrong. Aim to be level-headed. Are you a Psychology enthusiast but missed a bunch of psych-related questions? Don't discount them as silly mistakes or worse beat yourself up over them. Just go back and quickly review the topics, watch some videos, etc. Understand down to atomic detail why you didn't get that question by perpetually asking why (even if the deeper answer is something embarrassing like "*I didn't read this part because I was distracted by thinking about a question I didn't get last passage*"). We have seen many-a-nurse convince themselves that they don't need to review some specific topic, or lose morale from not getting a question they "*should*" have gotten because of X or Y experience. It's okay to fail, this is a system, and to win in the long run we can control our emotions. Here are some additional guidelines for this practice phase:

By the end of this phase, you should have gone through 300 questions of practice tests and 30 questions per day (*minimum*) in the High Content Phase and significantly more during your High Practice Phase.

Optional: Practice Test 4-5

More practice tests are optional. For example, doing 5 practice tests would mean doing an initial practice test, then 2 practice tests at the mid and endpoint of each phase. However this could easily be too exhaustive, particularly because of the detailed reflections will have to do to facilitate your improvement. Know yourself. If you suffer from severe testing anxiety, or deviated significantly from your study schedule, then consider this option. It's important to reiterate that getting yourself comfortable within an NCLEX testing environment and the "worst" case, stressful scenario is key. If you don't, you are at risk of making bad decisions that we have identified are the single greatest cause of failure for our students.

A Week Before Test Day

Once it is a week from test day, no more practice tests or questions. This may again depend on the tightness of your schedule, but give yourself at least 72 hours before test day for this. At this point, prioritize reviewing strong content areas and safety fundamentals so they are fresh. By the time it hits a day before the exam, rest. Do some light work if you feel like it, but not out of anxiety that you *need* to do it. No matter how you feel about your preparation, execution, etc... You deserve to relax and de-stress so you can be successful on the big day.

Test Day Tips

Sleep, sleep, sleep: If you take away anything, get to bed early the night before (earlier than you usually do). We do not care if you can "survive on 4" or want to do some last minute review... Go to bed. If you are having trouble use supplements or prescribed medication that you have used consistently before. Do not be testing anything new the night before. Remember this exam is literally designed to throw you off and mess with your head, and you need a stable foundation to counter that.

- **Be prepared, obviously:** The night before, put out clothes that you generally wore during your studying and practice exams, phone, water, ear-plugs, snacks and whatever else you need. For snacks, we recommend healthy snacks/sandwiches and a treat for when you finish the exam.

- **Try if you like:** We some success some little strategies to reduce nerves: cover the question counter with a small piece of tape; arrive early to the testing center to feel familiar with the area; eat a good breakfast and watch your favorite TV show; as silly as it might sound, take a long deep breath when you feel nerves getting to you.

- **Take a break:** You are not cool for not taking a break. Use the bathroom, eat some food. Even a simple location change for no particular reason can allow you to better reset for the next section.

- **When it's done, it's done:** Once the exam is over, relax. Thinking over what you got right or wrong should last less than 5 minutes. After that it's over. Have a treat if you brought one, or get a treat or reward from somewhere. You deserve it!

How Does This Book Fit Into Your Plan?

Now that we have outlined a bulletproof template to your NCLEX studies, let's see how this book can fit into this template and why. Note that these are how we observed the book used among graduates of nursing programs studying for the NCLEX, some of whom continue to use it as a reference in their nursing practice.

Insight #1: Use this book as an index for timed practice quizzes

We have tested the use of mnemonics in many forms. We unexpectedly found that a book is more useful than we thought. Why? If you use it in practice, flipping through pages quickly, you can find and reinforce your memory of mnemonics you need to answer questions. Thus, we recommend using this during timed practice quizzes in your everyday practice. We do not recommend doing this on practice tests, only practice quizzes. Practice tests should be closed-source and replicate the exam-environment so you can accurately gauge how you are performing and pat yourself on the back for making improvements under real test conditions.

Nevertheless, while doing the timed practice passages try to recall mnemonics yourself. Write down any you think of as soon as you have skimmed a question and determined pertinent topics. If you can't think of any, quickly flip through this book to see if any of them are relevant. If you are stuck on a *specific* question trying to recall specific information, also flip through this book. If you can't find any, note this question down. Once done with a passage and grading, look at the explanation of answers (if you have them). If you marked down the question already, or feel like you made a simple, silly mistake as you read the explanation, chances are this is where a simple mnemonic or memory tool could have helped you.

So, use a blank page in the book to brainstorm something memorable. If you feel like the explanation proved you made a more complex mistake, this should be a signal do look back at your content/research, and see if you can also make a mnemonic related to information (this is because the pain of that bigger mistake can influence you to recall memory even better the next time, given you still do some content review like we said earlier). We have also found that some students altered their study strategy, doing content for one topic but practice questions for the topic they studied yesterday, giving them a buffer to see if they could recall mnemonics well. Try this strategy and see if it works for you.

Insight #2: Take the book everywhere, if you can

This is fairly necessary if you are studying for this exam under a relatively busy schedule. If you have a job with low workload or free time, than this should be mandatory. A lot of people who succeed under these circumstances especially need to siphon free time and bring portable study materials: this book, flashcards, notes, etc. Then, do practice questions on a phone/tablet.

Insight #3: Abuse every page

This is less common among people who used this book, but those who did had the most positive impact on their score and their outlook towards using the book. For example, successful students actively scribbled or even ripped out pages they didn't need, wrote and thought about more creative, personal mnemonics and compiled them within this book. Some also took mnemonics from here and merely copied them into paper/online flashcards and did well. However, be systematic about using the latter, don't let the deck get too long. Alternatively, we used Post-it notes as flashcards and pasted them onto the blank pages of each section. This helps keep the book convenient and memory tactile. Meanwhile, it also forces you to distill important concepts down so you don't completely overload the book's space.

The Ultimate Goal

We hope that you have found our study plan template, as well as how to use this book within that plan helpful. Our realization is that there is a simple, criminally underrated strategy that allows us to game the NCLEX to pass as efficiently as possible. It's simple: this test is always a safety game, and critical thinking right after. If we simply allocate more time to building the right encyclopedia of memory shortcuts, we can save the time it takes to recall specific information and allocate time to questions that require more mental effort. It can even be fun, light practice that you can do in the downtime of a busy schedule where you can't go hardcore-library-study-mode. The goal is to treat your brain like an emotional computer. As you prepare, you allow yourself to search for mnemonics or memory tools you have strong meaning or emotions attached to. This key unlocks further memory tools on the blank pages, so you have a population of memory tricks around which to attack each question. It's not easy. It's never perfect. But in the long-run, from the NCLEX and beyond, you will notice the difference, even as you encounter real-life cases.

Next Tasks

Now that you have an idea about a study plan and how this book could be useful as you study for the NCLEX, we recommend some basic planning and reflection strategies. First, come up with a **5 Principle Study Plan**. It should not be as specific as we described earlier, that will require proper organization and scheduling tools (but you can write specific notes on the next page. As you take your practice tests, we also recommend **Reflections** after each to distill weaknesses, reflect on your emotions, and keep yourself aware and accountable. Let's go.

5 Principle Study Plan

1.

2.

3.

4.

5

Tip: Write in pencil so you can make small refinements later! Another tip: If you are anxious to start and tend to overwork yourself, make your 5th principle about how you will **rest**. If you are a little depressed about the prospect of starting and tend to procrastinate, give yourself some kind words on how/why you will **commit** to the study plan.

Additional Plan Notes:

Reflections

<u>Practice Test 1</u>:

<u>Practice Test 2</u>:

Reflections

Practice Test 3:

Practice Test 4:

Practice Test 5:

Care Assessment & Management

Management of Care Process

A Delicious PIE

A	**Assessment** The beginning of the nursing process where you will assess the patient holistically.
D	**Diagnosis:** After completing the assessment, you will put together an idea of what may be causing a problem for your patient.
P	**Planning** Together, the medical team will create a long-term action guide for the patient to achieve wellness.
I	**Implementation** This is where you will assist the patient in understanding and completing the action guide created by the medical team.
E	**Evaluation** After the allotted time frame, the patient will return for you to reassess the treatment plan's effectiveness.

Health Assessment Criteria

SAMPLE

S — Symptoms

What is your patient currently experiencing that is out of the ordinary?

A — Allergies

What allergies is your patient aware of? Have they had recent exposure?

M — Medications

What medications or treatments are currently being taken?

P — Past medical history

Does your patient have a past history of these symptoms or related diagnoses? What illnesses run in their family?

L — Last oral intake of medication

When was the last time they had any type of oral treatment? (also, when was their last meal?)

E — Events leading up to the illness or injury

What occurred before experiencing these symptoms?

Tip: Getting an incomplete and/or incorrect history is an extreme safety risk, and one of the most systemically common issues in medical practice. Complete information gathering is important in all conditions, even the highest-immediacy emergency such as in major trauma pre-op care.

Case Management Process

SAS-PIF-TCE ("sass, piff, teecee")

S	Screening
A	Assessing
S	Stratifying Risk
P	Planning
I	Implementing (Care Coordination)
F	Following-up
T	Transitioning (Transitional Care)
C	Communicating Post-Transition
E	Evaluation

Rights of Delegation

Right: CPCS

C (Right) Circumstance
consider patient setting, available resources, and task predicability/risk

P (Right) Person
delegating to healthcare person with correct scope

C (Right) Communication
give clear, concise, complete, and correct information. Describe objective, limits, and expectations

S (Right) Supervision
continue to monitor, evaluate, and intervene as needed

RN Scope Of Practice

IV ATE

IV	IV medications
A	Assesment
T	Teaching
E	Evaluate

RN has a well defined scope of practice relative to the role of LPN. One of primary importance in the exam context is that only RN (and physician) are able to administer IV medication. In practice, LPNs must be thoroughly trained to administer IV medication to a limited extent based on state laws (Nurse Practice Act) and facility rules. Even then, certain tasks like IV push, mixing IV solutions, or other blood product admin. are out of scope for LPNs.

More abstractly, the scope of an RN is to assess the client to establish nursing diagnosis, implement a plan of care, and evaluate results. The other goal is to teach other healthcare persons on the practice of nursing directly or through the management of care.

Safe Medication Administration Checklist

TRAMP

T — **Time**
Check the order to see when the patient's medication was last given.

R — **Route**
Verify which method their medication was administered.

A — **Amount**
How much does the patient need, and at what time intervals?

M — **Medication**
Make sure the name and order form are correct and check for possible errors.

P — **Patient**
Verify the patient's name and check their ID bracelet. Verify informed consent.

Tip: Note that this is very associated to the nurse's right of medication administration: (right) person, medication, dose, time, route, reason, documentation. You can use the mnemonic "My Patients Don't Really Take Real Drugs" to remember the first letter of each right.

5 R's Before Calling Physician

5 R's

R	Review patient assessment
R	Review vital signs
R	Review records: MAR, Labs, Recent Orders, Progress Notes
R	Review care pathway, policies and procedures
R	Ready relevant Information (e.g. chart, medication sheet, vital signs, code status, POLST, allergies)

Cheat Sheet

Care Assessment & Management

Care Fundamentals

AVPU Coma Scale

AVPU

A — **Alert**
The patient is awake, they can open their eyes voluntarily, and can move parts of their body.

V — **Voice**
They can respond vocally (even if only noises) or to a vocal stimulus (like a loud sound)

P — **Pain**
The patient reacts to pain stimuli (eg. sternum rub) by showing discomfort or reacting to injuries.

U — **Unresponsive**
There is no kind of reaction or response from the patient.

AVPU, a condensed version of the Glasgow Coma Scale (GCS), is used to assess a patient's consciousness based on their eye, vocal, and motor reactions. A is the top of the scale, whereas VPU are lower and indicate higher urgency for care.

Glasgow Coma Scale Reference

Eye Opening	Score
Spontaneous	4
To verbal command	3
To pain	2
No response	1
Verbal Response	
Oriented	5
Confused	4
Inappropriate words	3
Incomprehensible sounds	2
No response	1
Motor Response	
Obeys commands	6
Localizes pain	5
Withdraws from pain	4
Abnormal flexion (decorticate posturing)	3
Abnormal extension (decerebrate posturing)	2
No response	1
Total Score	
Mild TBI	13-15
Moderate TBI	9-12
Severe TBI	3-8

Pain Scale Reference

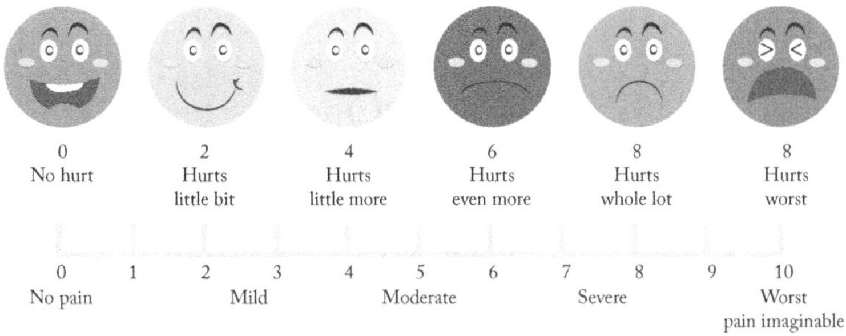

OPQRST Pain Assessment

OPQRST

O — Onset

"Did your pain start suddenly or gradually get worse and worse? What were you doing when pain started?"

P — Provokes or Palliates

"What makes your pain better or worse?"

Q — Quality

"What does your pain feel like?" (open-ended)

R — Radiates

"Point to where it hurts the most. Where does your pain go from there?"

S — Severity

"Rate pain from 1-10"

(helpful to provide references "1 means... 10 means..." or use face pain scale)

T — Time

"How long ago did pain start?"

All Vital Signs

P-THROB

P	Pain
T	Temperature
H	Heart Rate
R	Respirations
O	O_2 SATs
B	Blood Pressure

4H's of High Risk Signs

4H'S	
H	Has no pulse / breathless
H	Hemorrhage
H	Hypoglycemia
H	High Fever (>105)

Emergency Trauma Assessment

ABCDEFGHI
or ABCDEFG-Head-Toe-A**

A	Airway
B	Breathing
C	Circulation
D	Disability
E	Expose / Examine
F	Full set of Vitals
G	Give Comfort Measures
H	Head-to-Toe Assessment
I	Inspect Posterior

Trauma Types Assessment

DCAP-BTLS

D	Deformities
C	Contusions
A	Abrasions
P	Punctures/Penetrations
B	Burns
T	Tenderness
L	Lacerations
S	Swelling

Palpating Abdomen Assessment

Really Tough Girls Don't Cry

R	Rigidity
T	Tenderness
G	Guarding
D	Distention
C	Crepitus

ICP vs. Shock

ICP : "up, down, down, the wide streets"

↑ BP

↓ HR

↓ Respiratory rate

Widened pulse pressure

Shock : "down, up, up, the narrow alleys"

↓ BP

↑ HR

↑ Respiratory rate

Narrowed pulse pressure

Client In Traction Nursing Care

TRACTION

T Temperature
(Extremity, Infection)

R Ropes hang freely

A Alignment

C Circulation Check (5 P's)

T Type & Location of fracture

I Increase fluid intake

O Overhead trapeze

N No weights on bed or floor

IV Fluid Types

IHH

I	**Isotonic:** replaces fluid losses. 0.9% NS
H	**Hypotonic:** Pulls fulid into cells. 0,45% NS
H	**Hypertonic:** pulls fluid out of cells. 3% saline.

Environmental Health Assessment Checklist

I PREPARE

I	Investigate potential exposure
P	Present work/job-site
R	Residence
E	Environmental concerns
P	Past work/job-site
A	Activities
R	Referrals/resources
E	Educate

This is a common criteria of assessment for community health or public health nurses, and an aspect of any RNs scope of care (environmental safety). Typically human health hazards fall under the categories: housing, occupational, atmosphere, foodborne diseases, and waterborne diseases.

Family History Assessment

BALDCHASM

B	Blood pressure
A	Arthritis
L	Lung diseases
D	Diabetes
C	Cancers
H	Heart diseases
A	Alcoholism
S	Stroke
M	Mental health disorders

This mnemonic can be used to remember how to assess a patient's family medical history for genetically transmitted diseases, medical disorders, and chronic illnesses.

Circulatory Checks

5 P's

P Pain

P Paresthesia
sensation of numbness/tingling

P Paralysis

P Pulse
check for abnormal pulse amplitude
(radial, dorsalis pedis, and posterior tibial)

P Pallor
paleness or other deviation from skin tone

Minor Soft Tissue Injury Treatment

RICE

R	**Rest** Protect the injured area and rest as much as possible. Avoid putting weight on area for 48–72 hours
I	**Ice** Apply ice or a cold pack ASAP
C	**Compression** Wrap injured area with elastic bandage
E	**Elevation** Prop up the injured area

RICE can provide helpful criteria for treating sprains/strains and other soft-tissue injuries in a first-aid context. New research suggests that Rest is the most important for such injuries, and that Ice may not be as necessary. Additionally, avoiding anti-inflammatory medication and slowly introducing exercise after the Rest period can improve recovery processes

Blood Type Compatibility

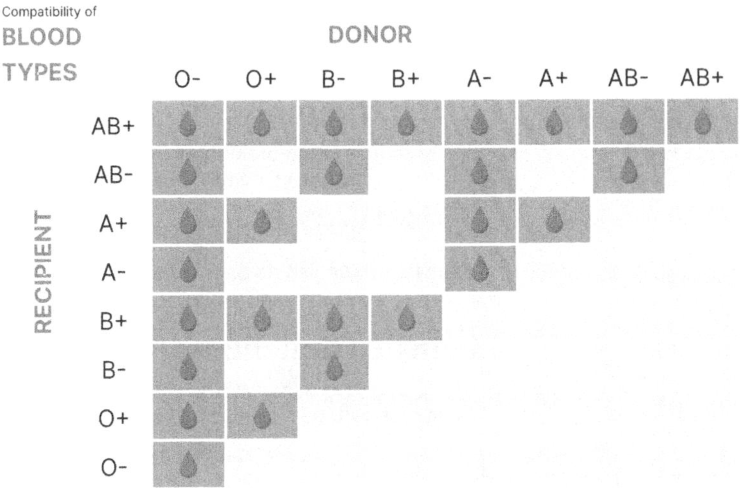

Most hospitals only give RNs the scope to perform blood transfusions due to extensive training. Key criteria for a transfusion:

- **prep completely** (blood typing: ABO, Rh factors; consent; history of past transfusions/reactions;)

- **give blood within 30 min of receiving from bank/la**b (complete full verification, vitals, other protocol)

- **fully infused in at most 4 hours**

- **if there is a reaction, stop immediately.**

Blood Transfusion Reactions

i HAF blood

H — Hemolytic

immune system is killing the donors RBCs due to mistyping, deadly

A — Allergic Reaction

immune system reacts to proteins from donor, anaphylaxis

F — Febrile (non-hemolytic)

recipient WBCs fighting donor WBCs, antibody buildup, common with past tranfusion history

Other rarer reactions that can occur are,

- **Septicemia**: infection enters the bloodstream and spreads (typically if transfusion started/ended late)

- **Graft-versus-host Disease**: deadly, delayed reaction (multiple days/weeks) where donor's T lymphocytes engraft onto recipient marrow, attacking tissues and causing immune response.

- **Blood contamination**: Hep B/C, HIV, etc. This is rare due to blood donor screening.

- **Circulatory or iron overload**: circulatory can cause acute respiratory distress (typically fluid leakage into lunds). Iron can accumulate and damage the liver, heart, etc. Both have higher likelihood with past transfusion history.

Activities of Daily Living (ADLs)

BATTED

B	Bathing
A	Ambulation walking or maneuvering around a space
T	Toileting
T	Transfers moving from a seated or reclined position
E	Eating
D	Dressing

Canes and Walkers

COAL and WWAL

C	Cane
O	Opposite
A	Affected
L	Leg (ie. on the stronger leg)
W	Walker
W	With
A	Affected
L	Leg

Prevention of Thrombophlebitis

6 E's

E	Early ambulation
E	Exercise
E	Elastic stockings
E	Elevate legs
E	Encourage fluids
E	Extend knees

Thrombophlebitis is a condition where a thrombus,or a blood clot, forms in a vein and can cause pain and inflammation. It can affect veins near the skin's surface or deeper veins, but it most commonly occurs in the legs and pelvis.

Key characteristics to consider for history are recent surgeries, prolonged immobility, obesity, smoking, family history of clotting, hormonal contraceptive use and pregnancy. Key characteristics of assessment are physical exams for edema/tenderness, D-dimer labs, venous doppler ultrasound, and additional pulmonary or neurovascular assessments.

Diet for Diarrhea/ Dehydration

BRAT

B	Banana
R	Rice
A	Applesauce
T	Toast

BRAT stands for the diet treatment for nonchronic diarrhea or severe dehydration. Nursing students may recall this is typically a short-term diet, as it is low in nutrients but easy to digest (producing less stool). More food items fit this category, but certain foods should be excluded such as:

- milk and dairy

- proteins like steak, pork, and salmon

- raw veggies, acidic fruits

- non-room-temperature drinks, alcohol, caffeine, or other stimulants of gut motility

Foods To Avoid With Celiac Disease

BROW

B	Barley
R	Rye
O	Oats (non-gluten-free)
W	Wheat

In celiac disease, an immune response forms against gluten, specifically gliadin, generating antibodies that damage small intestine mucosa (innermost lining). This leads to common GI symptoms, fatty stool, and malabsorption leading to long-term malnutrition.

Barley, Rye, Oats, and Wheat are all grains that should be avoided for those with Celiac disease (and considered for those with non-celiac gluten sensitivity). Importantly, wheat derivative products (of which there are many), malt, triticale, and brewer's yeast should also be avoided.

Substances To Avoid With Kidney Disease

limit Pro-Pho-Po-So-Flo

Pro	Proteins
Pho	Phosphates
Po	Potassium
So	Sodium
Flo	Fluids

Patients with diseased kidneys cannot easily maintain the body's fluid balance particularly with low urine output. In addition, clients with diseased kidneys must prevent buildup of waste products that a healthy renal system would typically filter. Thus, a diet program for conditions like Chronic Kidney Disease involve limiting consumption of proteins, potassium, sodium, phosphates (and phosphorus in dairy products).

Tip: Note that a common regimen for clients with diseased kidneys is consistent weighing to monitor fluid retention, monitoring for hyperkalemia, and CBC/EPO/creatinine labs.

Devices: Chest Tubes Management

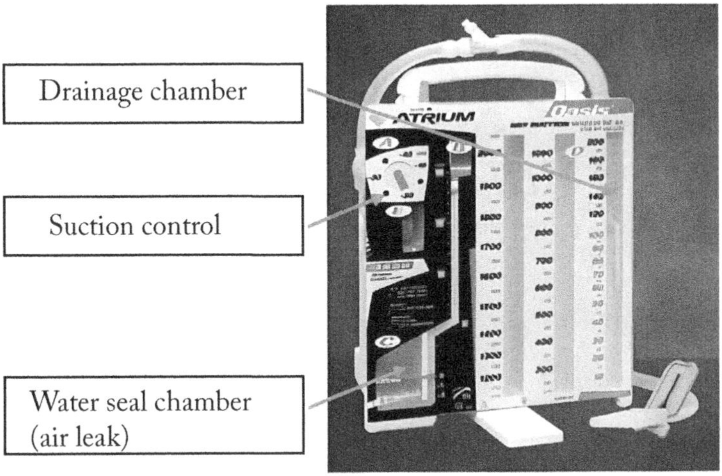

Establish negative pressure

Bubbling in water seal = air leak

Devices: Tracheostomy Tubes

OD

O	Obturator, ambu bag, suction, correct trach size
D	Decannulation: call rapid response, lay supine, provide oxygen (bag valve mask)

Devices: ECG Leads

WCSM

W — White to the right

C — Clouds over grass
(white over green)

S — Smoke over fire
(black over red)

M — My stomach loves chocolate
(brown on stomach)

Devices: Ventilator Alarms

HOLD

H	High Alarm
O	Obstruction due to increased secretions, kink, coughing or gagging
L	Low Pressure Alarm
D	Disconnection or leak in ventilator or in airway cuff or patient stops spontaneous breathing ("high...kink, low...leak")

Cheat Sheet

Care Fundamentals

Safety & Infection Control

Putting on / Taking off PPE

You drive to a fancy celebrity dinner...

Put on the dress (gown)...

Then your lipstick (mask)...

Then your shades (goggles)...

Lastly, your fancy driving (gloves)

You drive home from dinner...

Turn off the car (gloves)...

Then take your shades off (goggles)...

Once inside, you take off the dress (gown)...

Lastly, wipe off your lipstick (mask)

Procedure: Contact, Droplet, Airborne

Contact	"Cover ya hands (gloves) and body (gown), and Clean everything!" (clean and disinfect equipment or use dedicated/disposable equipment)
Droplet	"Cover ya whole face! (mask, goggles)"
Airborne	"Cover ya mouth (N95 or higher respirator) and Close the door!" (close off space)

Transmission Precautions: Airborne

Some Chickens Might Have TB

S	SARS
C	Chickenpox (varicella)
M	Measles
H	Herpes zoster (shingles)
TB	Tuberculosis

Transmission Precautions: Droplets

S-S-S-P-P-PIDER-M-M-M-An

S	Sepsis
S	Sscarlet fever
S	Streptococcal pharyngitis
P	Parvovirus b19
P	Pertussis
P	Pneumonia
I	Influenza
D	Diptheria (pharyngeal)
E	Epiglottitis
R	Rubella
M	Mumps
M	Meningitis
M	Myoplasma or Meningeal pneumonia
An	Adenovirus

Transmission Precautions: Contact

MRS. WEE

M	Multidrug resistant organism
R	RSV
S	Skin infections
W	Wound infections
E	Eenteric infections - C. diff.
E	Eye infections

Bleeding Precautions

RANDI

R	Razor Electric/Blades
A	Anticoagulants (blood thinners)
N	Needles-small gauge
D	Decrease needle sticks
I	Injury (Protect from)

Minor Bleeding Forms

BEEP

B	Bleeding gums
E	Epistaxis, also known as nose bleeds
E	Ecchymosis, also known as bruising
P	Petechiae

Hepatitis Transmission

I EAt Hepatitis

For types of hepatitis, remember I EAt Hepatitis. This is because Hep A and E contaminate through the fecal-oral route, typically through contaminated food and water. Whereas other types of Hepatitis (B, C, D) contaminate through parenteral contact with infected body fluids.

Risk of Infection Precautions

CCNNSND

C Close down

C Close down space

N No organisms

N No sick visitors or personnel

S Strict hand hygiene (no germs)

N No fresh food or plants

D Disinfect equipment

These are precautions for any client with a high risk of infection or is otherwise immunocompromised. A common presentation of this is Neutropenia, a condition where client has low white blood cell count (WBC < 1000, Neutrophil < 500). This triggers neutropenic precautions described above.

Cheat Sheet

Safety & Infection Control

OB & Maternity

Quick Tips

Expected Date of Delivery

LMP-3(mo.)+7(days)

The expected date of delivery (due date) is approximately the last menstrual period (LMP) plus 9 months and 7 days. If the LMP is not in the first few months of the year you can subtract 3 months and add 7 days from the LMP to get the same due date result for the next year.

Average Weight Gain / BMI

BMI: 18.5-24.99
(avg. 30lb weight gain)

Pregnancy Signs and Likelihood

M

"Maybe"

enlarged breasts, increased urination frequency, feeling of quickening (movement in uterus by fetus, however this actually happens at 16-20 weeks)

B

"Probably"

period stops, positive pregnancy test, chadwick's sign (cyanosis of cervix), goodell's sign (softening of cervix)

C

"Certainly"

fetal heart tones detected, fetal skeleton detected

Prenatal Care Checklist

ABCDEF

A	Amniotic fluid?
B	Bleeding?
C	Contractions?
D	Dysuria?
E	Edema?
F	Fetal movement?

Questions to ask about Prenatal Care can be remembered very simply with the alphabet! Use A-F to ask these questions: ABCDEF. These are the most commonly asked questions for pregnant women. The answers to them determine if tests need to be ordered, and if so, what kind.

Womb/Fundus Progression

"puberty"

12 weeks
can palpate fundus

"graduated umb. college"

22 weeks
fundus at the umbilical

"working for cash money (cm)"

>24 weeks
fundal height (cm) should be about equal to number of weeks.

Stages of Labor Reference

Stage 1: Cervix dilates from 0-10cm

- *Latent phase:* 1-3cm dilated. Contractions 5-30min apart (can happen for days to weeks)
- *Active phase:* 4-7cm dilated. Contractions 3-5min apart
- *Transition phase:* 8-10cm dilated, Contractions 2-3min apart
- Note: contractions >90sec or <2min apart is dangerous (possible fetal hypoxia)

Stage 2: Delivery of Baby

Stage 3: Delivery of Placenta

Stage 4: Postpartum

Common Pregnancy Medications:
If a patient is pre-term and having contractions, slow down contractions with tocolytic drugs. (commonly terbutaline or magnesium sulfate, but no specific drug approved for this purpose)

If patient is past her due date and induced labor required: use oxytocin or pitocin (also used to control postpartum hemorrhage)

Pregnancy Complications:

- Placenta previa
- Eruptio placentae
- Pre-eclampsia
- Eclampsia

Interventions for Labor & Delivery Complications

LION Pee

L	Left side
I	Increase IV
O	Oxygenate
N	Notify physician
P	Pitocin (oxytocin) (note: follow clear protocol and dual verification before admin)

Severe Preeclampsia: HELLP Syndrome

HELLP

H	Hemolysis (destruction of red blood cells)
E	Elevated
L	Liver enzymes and
L	Low
P	Patelet count

Abdomial Pain in Pregnant Patients: Possible Causes

LARA CROFT

L	Labor
A	Abruptio Placenta
R	Rupture (e.g., ectopic/uterine rupture)
A	Abortion (Spontaneous)
C	Cholestasis
R	Rectus sheath hematoma (RSH)
O	Ovarian tumor
F	Fibroids
T	Torsion of the uterus

Fetal Heart Rate Change Causes

VEAL
CHOP

This nursing mnemonic indicates different fetal heart rate changes and the causes behind them during earlier stages of pregnancy, such as during nonstress tests. (Fetal HR of 110-160)

Variable decelerations → Cord compression

- Variable decelerations could indicate that the fetus's blood supply is limited. Because the fetus receives blood supply through the umbilical cord to receive oxygen, this suggests the cord is compressed. The decelerations are unpredictable and can impact heart rate, causing frequent drops. Some possible causes include:
    - The mother and fetus's positioning
    - True knot in the umbilical cord
    - Nuchal cord entanglements
    - Insufficient amniotic fluid
    - Rupture of the uterus
    - Umbilical cord prolapse
- Adjusting the mother's position to alleviate umbilical cord compression may manage this, however further exams and treatment include: examining the cervix to check for cord issues, administering an IV to increase blood volume, administering oxygen, or in extreme cases prep for cesarean birth.

Early deceleration → Head compression

- With early decelerations, the heart rate slows progressively before the contraction reaches its peak. This typically occurs when the baby's head is compressed.
- This either occurs during any onset of uterine contractions and in later stages of labor as the baby's head descends through... ...the birth canal (both usually harmless). But, it can also be a more serious issue with preterm or transverse babies during premature labor.

continued →

- Changing the mother's position to increase the flow of oxygen may reduce compression and alleviate early deceleration. For instance, having the mother lie down on their left side with their knees into their chest can reduce pressure on the vena cava (the large vein carrying blood from the heart) to provide sufficient blood to the uterus. Ongoing fetal heart rate monitoring is also advised.

Accelerations → OK

- Fetal heart rate accelerations are temporary increases of 15 bpm or more lasting 15 seconds or more. These changes are natural and healthy, indicating that the fetus is getting sufficient oxygen.

- Spontaneous accelerations should occur during birth, but doctors may try to trigger them if none occur naturally. The following interventions may be used:
    - Placing a finger on the baby's head through the cervix
    - Gently rocking the mother's abdomen
    - Providing vibroacoustic stimulation (a short burst of sound)

Late decelerations → Placental insufficiency (use "LION Pee" Protocol)

- Late decelerations occur when the fetal heart rate gradually decreases for 30 seconds or more after a contraction. This change is the most concerning of all as it suggests placental insufficiency, which could lead to serious issues such as shortage of oxygen for the baby.

- As with early decelerations, one immediate intervention may be turning the patient on their side and having them bring their knees to their chest to increase blood flow. If the issue persists, interventions such as an oxygen mask, intravenous hydration, and cesarean birth may be needed.

APGAR Newborn Health Score

APGAR

A — Appearance
Is the baby blue/pale, blue/pink, or pink?

P — Pulse
Is the pulse absent, under 100, or greater than 100?

G — Grimace
Response to stimulation

A — Activity
Flexing of the limbs

R — Respiration
Is there crying and is it weak or strong?

The APGAR score is used to gauge the health of a baby at 1-5 minutes after being born. The following reference highlights the point system used to score from 0-10:

SCORE	0 points	1 point	2 points
Appearance (Skin color)	Cyanotic / Pale all over	Peripheral cyanosis only	Pink
Pulse (Heart rate)	0	<100	100-140
Grimace (Reflex irritability)	No response to stimulation	Grimace or weak cry when stimulated	Cry when stimulated
Activity (Tone)	Floppy	Some flexion	Well flexed and resisting extension
Respiration	Apneic	Slow, irregular breathing	Strong cry

Postpartum Assessment/Care Criteria

BUBBLE HER

B	Breasts
U	Uterus
B	Bowels
B	Bladder
L	Lochia
E	Episiotomy, which also includes C-section incisions or other lacerations
H	Homan's sign
E	Emotional Status
R	Respiratory System

The BUBBLE HER mnemonic device can help you provide patients who have given birth with proper postpartum assessments and care. This memory trick is designed to help you remember the specific areas that will need examination.

Assessment Tests For Fetal Well-Being

ALONE

A	Amniocentesis
L	L/S ratio (1.8:1>)
O	Oxytocin Challenge Test
N	Non-Stress Test
E	Estriol (E3) Level

The following assessment tests are common ways to assess fetal well-being. Amniocenesis uses extracted amniotic fluid from the abdomen to assess genetic conditions like Down Syndrome.

Lecithin-to-sphingomyelin (L/S) ratio assess levels of two lung surfactants that show how mature lung development is (1.8:1 ratio or higher indicates maturity).

Oxytocin challenge test (OCT) evaluates fetal tolerance to uterine contractions (ie. will the baby stay healthy when the client is in labor). Non-stress test is a passive test of fetal heart rate in response in relation to contractions or fetal movement.

Estriol level is checked around week 15-20, as it is a marker of fetal growth (as it signals growth of the uterus) and progression towards labor. Low levels are a sign of fetal demise, congenital abnormalities, or genetic hormonal disorders like Down Syndrome

Fetal Positions

Safe: Head Tucked First (LOA/ROA)
Danger: Sideways or Booty First

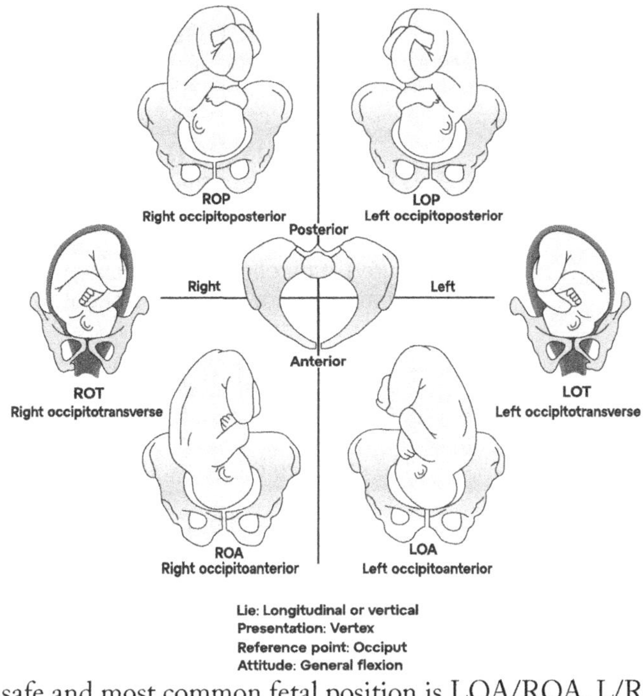

The safe and most common fetal position is LOA/ROA. L/R is left/right. O is occiput, referring the bone at back of fetus head faces out (ie. fetus head is "tucked in"). A is anterior, meaning facing the base of pelvis (ie. fetus face is "on the pillow"). This is safe because the head, the largest part to pass, starts out smaller in diameter, which helps match the dilation of the cervix. Thus, any breech positions (ie. booty first) are always more dangerous, increasing likelihood of umbilical cord prolapse, hypoxia, and postpartum hemorrhage. This position in addition to transverse (ie. sideways positions, not pictured here but virtually impossible to deliver) will often require C-Section or other assistance.

Induction of Labor: Bishop Score

DPECS

D — **Dilation**
Measured in centimeters, dilation describes how widened the cervix has become.

P — **Position**
This describes the position of the baby.

E — **Effacement**
Measured in percentage, effacement is a measurement of how thin and elongated the cervix is.

C — **Consistency**
Ranging from firm to soft, this describes the consistency of the cervix. The softer the cervix, the closer to delivering the baby.

S — **Station**
Fetal Station is the measurement of how far baby's head descends into pelvis relative to the ischial spines. (range from -5 to +5)

Reference Bishop Score Table

Score	Cervix dilation	Cervix effacement	Fetal station	Cervix position	Cervix consistency
0	closed	0% to 30%	-3	posterior	firm
1	1-2 cm	4% to 50%	-2	mid-position	moderately firm
2	3-4 cm	60% to 70%	-1	anterior	soft
3	5+ cm	80% or greater	+1	anterior	soft

Young Children Pain Scale

	FLACC Scale	0	1	2
1	Face	No particular expression or smile	Occasional grimace or frown, withdrawn, disinterested	Frequent to constant from, clenched jaw, quivering chin.
2	Legs	Normal position or relaxed	Uneasy, restless, tense	Kicking or legs drawn up.
3	Activity	Lying quietly, normal position, moves easily.	Squirming, shifting back and forth, tense.	Arched, rigid or jerking.
4	Cry	No crying (awake or asleep)	Moans or whimpers: occasional complaint.	Crying steadily, screams or sobs, frequent complaints.
5	Consolability	Content, relaxed.	Reassured by occasional touching, hugging or being talked to, distractable.	Difficult to console or comfort.

Fetal Distress during Induced Labor

Stop MOAN

S	STOP infusion (of uterine stimulant)
M	Mom turned on the Notify Provider side
O	O_2 administration
A	Assess baby and mom to see if changes occurred
N	Notify Provider

Post-Episiotomy Healing Evaluation

REEDA

R	Redness
E	Edema
E	Ecchymosis
D	Discharge, Drainage
A	Approximation

Redness with pain, excess edema, ecchymosis (bruising), or discharge/drainage from the wound can all be signs of problems with healing after an episiotomy. Wound edges should be well approximated. Topical ointments and ice packs may be indicated if there is pain or excess swelling, or other signs of infection.

Probable Signs of Pregnancy

CHOP BUGS

C	**Chadwicks** bluish discoloration of lower uterine segment
H	**Hegar** softening of lower uterine segment
O	**Outlining of Fetal Body**
P	**Positive pregnancy test** the presence of gonadotropin in urine
B	**Ballotement** sinking and rebound of the fetus
U	**Uterine Enlargement** at 12 weeks gestation felt just above symphysis pubis
G	**Goodells** Softening of the cervix
S	**Souffle, Contraction, and Braxton Hicks** (painless contraction at 28 weeks)

Cheat Sheet

OB & Maternity

Pediatrics & Development

Reference: Common Pediatric Milestones

1 month:
grasp reflex

4 months:
roll front to back, smile

6 months:
roll back to front, sounds, teeth erupt, can introduce solid food

8 months:
sits unsupported

9-12 months:
starting to walk

24 months:
kick ball, can use stairs

3 yrs:
runs, draws shapes

4 years:
uses scissors, can pour beverages

Tip: If you receive a question that asks you to check off what a child can do at X age, choose option(s) that are more guaranteed (eg. early milestone motor/fine-motor skills, or physical processes like teeth eruption are more predictably "on-time" than social skills)

Congenital Heart Defect (Tetralogy of Fallot)

The blood isn't oxygenating at VORP speed

V	Ventricular Septal Defect
O	Overriding Aorta
R	Right Ventricular Hypertrophy
P	Pulmonary Outflow Tract Obstruction

Pediatric Hypoxia Symptoms

FINES

F	Feeding difficulty
I	Inspiratory Stridor
N	Nares Flares
E	Expiratory Grunting
S	Sternal Retractions

Psychosocial

Symptoms of Mania

DIG FAST

D	Distractibility
I	Indiscretion/excessive with pleasurable activities
G	Grandiosity
F	Flight of ideas
A	Activity increase
S	Sleep deficit decrease in the need for sleep
T	Talkativeness

In addition, mania is commonly one of the primary symptoms of bipolar disorder. It can also be the side effect from the use of prescription medications as well as some illicit drugs.

5 A's of Alzheimer's Disease

5 A's

A — **Amnesia**
loss of memory

A — **Anomia**
difficulty thinking of words

A — **Apraxia**
difficulty producing speech

A — **Agnosia**
difficulty identifying objects/people in 1 or more senses

A — **Aphasia**
inability to express or understand spoken/written language

Altered Mental State Possible Causes

AEIOU TIPS

A	Alcohol
E	Epilepsy/Electrolytes
I	Insulin/Inborn errors of metabolism
O	Overdose/Oxygen
U	Uremia
T	Trauma
I	Infection
P	Psychiatric/Poisoning
S	Stroke/Subarachnoid Hemorrhage

Signs of Parkinson's Disease

TRAP

T — **Tremor**
involuntary, rhythmic shaking or twitching of one or more parts of the body

R — **Rigidity**
muscle stiffness (commonly in face)

A — **Akinesia**
loss of ability to move muscles voluntarily

P — **Postural instability**
difficulty balancing, unsteady standing/walking

Psychiatric Patients Management Criteria

SLTM-LessR

S	Safety
L	(Setting) Limits
T	(Establishing) Trusting relationship
M	Medications
LessR	Less Restrictive methods/environment

Alcohol/Drug Addiction Screening

CAGE

C Cut down

A Annoyed

G Guilty

E Eye opener

The CAGE-AID Questionnaire

1) Have you ever felt that you ought to Cut down on your drinking or drug use?

2) Have people Annoyed you by criticizing your drinking or drug use?

3) Have you ever felt bad or Guilty about your drinking or drug use?

4) Have you ever had a drink or use drugs first thing in the morning to steady your nerves or to get rid of a hangover? (ie. as an eye opener)

If a client responds yes to 2 or more of these questions, they are considered to have clinically significant evidence for Alcohol Use Disorder or Substance Abuse Disorder.

Sudden Altered Mental Status (AMS) Possible Causes

Psych MINDS

Psych	**Psychiatric** (Psychosis, extreme depression. other)
M	**Metabolic** (Low water, oxygen, sugar, Na, Ca, thyroid)
I	**Infections** (UTI, encephalitis, meningitis, pneumonia)
N	**Nervous** (TBI, bleed, seizure, stroke)
D	**Drugs** (Prescription antiseizure/cholinergics, corticosteroids, sedatives, alcohol or opioid overdose/withdrawal)
S	**Shock** (cariogenic or other)

Note: Subcategories of AMS are Delirium (acute change in attention/cognition or sudden confusion; reversible), Psychosis (temporary disconnection from reality), and Dementia (irreversible progressive decline in mental function).

Dementia Possible Symptoms

DEMENTIA

D	Drug and alcohol use
E	Eyes and ears
M	Metabolic and Endocrine disorders
E	Emotional disorder
N	Neurologic disorders
T	Tumors and trauma
I	Infection
A	Arteriovascular disease

Depression Symptoms

SeLF WAH

S	Sadness
L	Lethargy
F	Fatigue
W	Weight Gain/Loss
A	Anhedonia (loss of pleasure in doing everyday activities)
H	Hallucinations/Delusions

Therapeutic Communication Techniques

AIO

A — Acknowledge
a patient's feelings or concerns

I — "I" Statements:
Do not say "you did this wrong" or "you should do this".

O — Open-ended questions:
"Tell me how you are feeling? Tell me more? Can you explain this?"

Opiod Effects

BAD AMERICANS

B	Bradycardia & hypotension
A	Anorexia
D	Diminished pupilary size
A	Analgesia
M	Miosis
E	Euphoria
R	Respiratory depression
I	Increased smooth muscle activity (biliary tract constriction)
C	Constipation
A	Ameliorate cough reflex
N	Nausea and vomiting
S	Sedation

Drug Withdrawal

upper→lower, downer→higher

On a stimulant (upper) and having withdrawal → they go low

Low HR/BP/RR, Fatigue, Depression

On a depressant (downer) and having withdrawal → they go high.

High HR/BP/RR, Tremors, N/V (nausea and vomiting), Irritability, Seizures, Diaphoresis (excessive sweating).

Common Stimulants:

- Caffeine
- Cocaine
- Metamphetamines
- Adderall

Common Depressants:

- Alcohol
- Benzodiazepines (eg. Xanax)
- Barbiturates

Cheat Sheet

Psychosocial

Topics: Endocrine

3 K's of Type 1 Diabetes

3K's	
K	Keep insulin nearby (insulin dependent)
K	Kids (adolescent onset)
K	Ketosis (DKA occurs in Type 1)

Hypothyroidism Symptoms

MOM'S SO TIRED

M	Memory loss
O	Obesity
M	Malar flush/Menorrhagia
S	Slowness (mentally and physically)
S	Skin and hair dryness
O	Onset gradual
T	Tiredness
I	Intolerance to cold
R	Really low BP
E	Energy levels fall
D	Depression/Delayed relaxation of reflexes

Type 1 Diabetes Symptoms

PTH

P	Peepee Polyuria - excessive urination
T	Thirsty Polygypsia - excessive thirst
H	Hungry Polyphagia - excessive appetite

Type 1 Diabetes Treatment

Don't DIE from Diabetes

D Diet

I Insulin
(continue to administer even if patient tends to feel sick)

E Exercise

3 A's of Type 2 Diabetes

3A's

A	Adult Onsent
A	Absent Ketones (No ketosis)
A	Avoid excess carbs and cals (from an unhealthy lifestyle)

Type 2 Diabetes Treatment

A DREAM

A — Anorectics
drugs that cause suppression of appetite (eg. semaglutide, GLP-1 agonists)

D — Diet
avoid excess carbs and cals

R — Resources
provide education on prevention and management

E — Exercise
at least 30min x 5 days a week

A — Additional Insulin as needed

M — Metformin
Oral hypoglycemic medication

Diabetes Insipidus

Insipidus → I-need-a-SIP-of-this

This rare chronic condition causes the body's fluids to become unbalanced, leading to excessive thirst and urination (I need a SIP of this water!) via decreased ADH

Symptoms of Diabetic Ketoacidosis

Diabetic Keto Acidosis

D	Dehydration
K	Ketones, K+ high, Kussmaul breathing
A	Acidosis, Acetone Breath (smells fruity)

Causes of Diabetic Ketoacidosis

5 I's

I	**Infection** Urinary, respiratory, skin
I	**Infarction** Myocardial infarction, stroke, bowel, bone, skin
I	**Infant on board (Pregnancy)**
I	**Indiscretion with diet or exercise** Non-compliance with diabetic diet (e.g., sugar, carbohydrates or alcohol) and exercise guidance
I	**Insulin (lack thereof)** Pump failure, skipping insulin doses (treatment is IV fluids with regular insulin admin.)

Hypoglycemia Treatment

74 (7D4)

70 — 70
Blood Glucose < 70

D — Drunk symptoms
slurred speech, delayed reaction time, increased HR/RR, decreased BP, cold

D — Drink Juice
(rapid high glycemic index carb intake)

D — Drug
Glucagon (injection)

D — Do less exercise
(or less insulin if patient already had recent insulin admin)

Insulin Administration

RIL

R — **Rapid acting insulin** like Lispro or Aspart has a 15-min onset, peaks at 30 min. (hence timing 30min before meals), and generally lasts 3 hours

I — **Intermediate acting insulin** like NPH has a 6 hour onset, peaks at 8 hrs, and generally lasts 12 hours

L — **Long acting insulin** like Lantus (glargine) has no peak and lasts 12-24hrs. This is given 1-2x per day… typically at the same time of day everyday near bedtime

"clear before cloudy"

For compound IV push (mixing insulin), it is useful to control client blood glucose throughout the day with one injection. To administer, regular rapid-acting insulin (clear) should be drawn into the syringe first, before the intermediate-acting NPH (cloudy). This prevents possible contamination from occurring. Administer 30 minutes before meals, and recall the full process of insulin administration:

"(air) cloudy, (air) clear, (draw) clear, (draw) cloudy"

Check order → Wash hands; gather and clean materials → Roll NPH vial → Draw air for NPH and push → Draw air for regular insulin and push → Actually draw regular insulin and check for air bubbles → Actually draw NPH and check for air bubbles. → Administer at the abdomen, upper buttocks, outer thigh, or back of upper arms

Symptoms of Hyperthyroidism

STING

S — Sweating

T — Tremors or Tachycardia

I — Intolerance to heat
Irregular period, Irritability, Irregular eyes (e.g., weakness or bulging)

N — Nervousness
Neurological (e.g., chorea, myopathy, paralysis)

G — Goitre
Gastrointestinal problems (such as vomiting, nausea, as well as constipation or diarrhea)

Topics: Neurology

Signs of a Stroke

FAST

F	Facial drooping
A	Arm weakness
S	Speech difficulty
T	Time to call emergency services, fast!

Note: FAST is an acronym used by the American Stroke Association, designed to help both medical and nonmedical personnel identify the signs of a stroke. Other signs include sudden confusion/denial, vision problems (eg. eye deviation), dizziness, and headache (with no known cause)

Multiple Sclerosis Symptoms

DEMYELINATION

D	Diplopia
E	Eye movement painful
M	Motor weakness and spasticity
Y	Ystagmus
E	Elevated temperature
L	Lhermitte's phenomenon
N	Neuropathic pain
A	Ataxia
T	Talking slurred
I	Impotence
O	Overactive Bladder
N	Numbness

Signs of Cholinergic Crisis

SLUDGE

S	Salivation / Sweating (Diaphoresis)
L	Lacrimation (tears)
U	Urinary (Incontinence)
D	Defecation / Diarrhea
G	Gastric upset
E	Emesis or vomiting

In a cholinergic crisis, the body fails to breakdown acetylcholine (ACh) properly, leading to excess ACh that overstimulates neuromuscular junction by continuously depolarizing post-synaptic membrane. Note that the above are more subtle signs. Other subtler signs are blurry vision, bradycardia, and flushed skin. More severe signs are seizures, flaccid muscle paralysis, and respiratory depression/failure. More severe presentation can have more specific causes like overdose of acetylcholinesterase inhibitors, and exposure to specific insecticides and nerve gases.

Topics: Renal

Enlarged Prostate Signs

Weren't FUN

W Weak
weak urine stream or difficulty starting

F Frequency
frequent rate of urination

U Urgency
increased urgency of urination

N Nocturia
increased urination frequency at night

An enlarged prostate often generates these signs/symptoms. These can worsen in severity over time, and lead to sudden inability to urinate, cause urinary tract infections and bladder/kidney damage. Assessment of the prostate typically involves a digital rectal exam to detect size, obtaining urine sample to rule out infection, and a blood test for Prostate-specific Antigen (PSA).

Topics: Hematology

Deep Vein Thrombosis Diagnosis

DVT

D Dilated veins / Discoloration

V Venography is gold standard

T Tenderness of thigh and calf

Deep Vein Thrombosis (DVT) is a blood clot that forms in a deep vein, usually in the leg (but sometimes pelvis/arm) that can cause serious injury or fatality. Pain, weakness, and discoloration in the affected area can be signs of DVT, however closer assessment of vein dilation and discoloration is a stronger sign. Typically tenderness of thigh and/or calf is the most common, and can categorize DVT into proximal DVT (thigh), which more likely to embolize and cause death, and distal DVT (calf), which is more isolated and treatable with anticoagulants and compression stockings. To picture and thus diagnose DVT, Venography — X-ray imaging of veins with dye —is instrumental. Although a less invasive imaging technique like duplex ultrasound can also be used.

3 V's of Clot Formation

3 V's

V	Venostasis slowed or stagnating blood flow
V	Vessel trauma (endothelial or vessel wall)
V	Viscosity of blood hypercoagulability

Also known as Virchow's Triad, these are commonly cited contributors to thrombosis (clot formation). Slowed or turbulent blood flow can cause buildup from periods of prolonged immobility like surgery or a long flight (think traffic on the highway). Damage to vessel walls can occur from surface injuries and internal coagulation onto foreign objects, bacteria, or medical devices (think construction on highway). Thickness of the blood itself, or high viscosity, can itself occur particularly from genetic mutation from coagulation factor, severe trauma/burn, cancer, smoking, obesity, and advanced age (think bigger trucks on the highway)

Topics: Cardiology

3 T's of Cyanotic Defects

3 T's

T	Tetralogy of Fallot
T	Truncus Arteriosus
T	Tricuspid Atresia

These are the defects of Cyanotic Heart Disease (CHD). This is the most common type of birth defect and leading cause of death in children with congenital malformations.

Heart Murmur Phases

hARD ASS MRS. MS. D

hARD	Aortic Regurg = Diastolic
ASS	Aortic Stenosis = Systolic
MRS.	Mitral Regurg = Systolic
MS. D	Mitral Stenosis = Diastolic

Heart Auscultation Areas Order

APE To Man

A — **Atrial**

Second intercostal space to the right of the sternum

P — **Pulmonic**

Second intercostal space to the left of the sternum

E — **Erb's point**

Third intercostal space to the left of the sternum, directly below the pulmonic area (Erb = 3 letters, 3rd in order)

T — **Tricuspid**

Fourth intercostal space to the left of the sternum

M — **Mitral**

Fifth intercostal space at the midclavicular line (below nipple line)

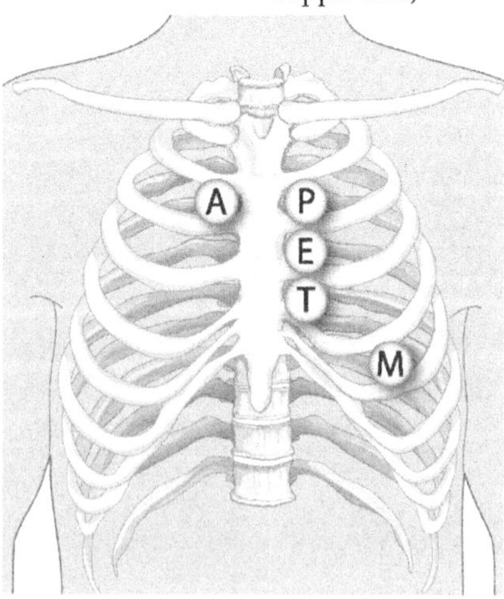

Signs of Endocarditis

FAM=E

F	Fever
A	Anemia
M	Murmur
E	Endocarditis

Endocarditis refers to the inflammation of the inner linings of the heart ("endo" = within/inside, "card" = heart, "itis" = inflammation). This is typically a rare, life-threatening infection of the inner lining from bacteria or fungi in the bloodstream. In developed countries, this is mostly from gram-positive streptococci, staphylococci, or enterococci. This causes symptoms of full body fever, anemia, chills, and possible heart murmur. While treatable with antibiotics, cases of more damage can require heart valve replacement surgery.

Acute Coronary Syndrome Test

BROW

R	Referred pain
U	Unexplained sweating
S	Shortness of breath
H	Heart Fluttering (with chest pain)

If someone satisfies the criteria for this test, they should visit a hospital as soon as possible. There, a professional can diagnose Acute Coronary Syndrome (ACS) via ECG and blood tests for cardiac biomarkers. This can help the ACS into Heart attack (either ST or non-ST segment elevation Myocardial Infarction (MI) via ECG reading) or unstable angina (No ECG or blood test indications.)

Possible Causes of Harmful Heart Murmur

SPAMS

S	Stenosis of a valve
P	Partial obstruction
A	Aneurysm
M	Mitral
S	Septal defect

Signs of Cor Pulmonale

Please Read His/Her Tricuspid

P	Peripheral edema
R	Raised jugular venous pressure (JVP)
H	Hepatomegaly
T	Tricuspid incompetence

This phrase is designed to help nurses identify cor pulmonale, which is a condition that causes the right side of the heart to fail.

Treatment of Congestive Heart Failure

UNLOAD FAST

U	Upright position
N	Nitrates
L	Lasix
O	Oxygen
A	Ace inhibitors
D	Digoxin
F	Fluid decrease
A	Afterload decrease
S	Sodium decrease
T	Test dig level, ABG, and K+ levels

Topics: Respiratory

Asthma Treatment

ASTHMA

A	Adrenergic (Albuterol)
S	Steroids
T	Theophylline
H	Hydration (IV)
M	Mask (Oxygen)
A	Antibiotics

Common Causes of Pulmonary Embolism

BAD FAT

B

Bacteria

A cause of bacterial embolism is when an area of the body becomes infected with bacteria, resulting in the formation of pus. These may become dangerous if dislodged from their original location. Like other emboli, a septic embolism may be fatal.

A

Air

Air can travel through the circulatory system and when in an artery, may directly stop blood flow to an area fed by the artery. Common causes of air emboli include surgery, trauma, scuba diving and being on a ventilator.

D

Deep Vein Thrombosis (DVT)

Pulmonary embolism most commonly occurs from thrombus formation which embolizes. A classic example of this is a DVT of the leg embolizing into the pulmonary arteries.

F

Fat

Fat emboli can occur from fracture of long bones, and are also associated with liposuction. A common exam question involves immobilized trauma patients developing fat embolisms.

A

Amniotic Fluid

Though rare and not completely understood, amniotic fluid can lead to pulmonary embolism. When amniotic fluid enters the mother's blood stream via the placental bed of the uterus and trigger an allergic reaction. This reaction then results in cardiorespiratory collapse.

T

Tumor

Embolism can also occur from tumors that have broken off and made their way into the bloodstream.

Detecting Epiglottitis

AIR RAID

A Airway closed

I Increased pulse

R Restlessness

R Retractions
(which nurses will observe when the muscles found in between the ribs pull inward as the patient breathes)

A Anxiety

I Increased inspiratory stridor
(the sound that air makes when the airflow through the larynx is turbulent)

D Drooling

Epiglottitis is the inflammation of the epiglottis, which can block the airway and cause client distress. Note that clients, particularly children, will report severe sore throat, pain while swallowing, and difficulty breathing, which are also positive indications of epiglottitis

6 P's of Shortness of Breath

6 P's

P Pulmonary bronchial constriction

P Possible foreign body

P Pulmonary embolism

P Pneumothorax

P Pump failure
Inability to pump enough blood ie. Congestive Heart Failure

P Pneumonia

Shortness of breath, or dyspnea, is characterized by feeling short of air or increased effort required to breathe or get enough air. There are 6 P's for common, dangerous reasons this may be the case. There are more mild, transient causes such as: heavy exercise, allergies, high altitude, tight clothing, and sedentary lifestyle. However, it is important to rule out the 6 P's first in a client care context.

Topics: Musculoskeletal & Integumentary

5 P's of Compartment Syndrome

5 P's

P	Pallor (pale skin tone)
P	Pain typically in lower leg/foot
P	(Faint) Pulse
P	Paralysis
P	Paresthesia abnormal feeling on skin eg. "pins and needles"

Compartment syndrome refers to too much pressure around the client's muscles (compartment), typically from internal bleeding or inflammation that then damages muscles and nerves. If compartment syndrome is detected after a traumatic incident is a medical emergency sometimes requiring surgery to remove the compressing tissue. More chronic conditions may also require this in severe cases, though typically rest and monitored exercise help.

Cleft Lip Post-op Care

CLEFT LIP

C	Choking precautions
L	Lie on back
E	Evaluate Airway
F	Feed Slowly
T	Teaching
L	Larger nipple opening
I	Incidence increased in males
P	Prevent crust formation and aspiration

Burns Criteria

SPF-TC

S	Superficial (1st degree): Redness, heat, pain, blanching, dry
P	Partial thickness (2nd degree): Wet, blisters pale, pink, pain.
F	Full thickness (3rd degree): Waxy, charred, pale, white, No pain/sensation.
T	**Treatment:** Fluids, Pain medications, Topical antibiotics, high caloric intake diet.
C	Calculating burns rule of 9

There are three degrees of burn: superficial, partial thickness, and full thickness (think SPF, like sunscreen). To calculate how much of the body is burned in % you can use the rule of 9. This divides the body into amounts that are 9% of the body's surface area, with some exceptions:

Front and back of the head and neck = 9%

Front and back of each arm and hand = 9% x 2 = 18%

Chest equals 9%

Stomach/abdomen = 9%

Upper and lower back = 9% x 2 = 18%

Front and back of each leg and foot for both legs = 18% x 2 = 36%

Genital area = 1%

Topics: Gastrointestinal

Appendicitis Signs

PAINS

P	Pain (RLQ)
A	Anorexia loss of appetite for food (not anorexia nervosa)
I	Increased temp (fever) and WBC (WBC: 15,000 – 20,000)
N	Nausea
S	Signs (McBurney's, Psoas)

Appendicitis is a medical emergency that occurs when the appendix becomes inflamed and swollen usually due to a blockage. This thereafter requires surgery and antibiotics to prevent rupture. Pain is usually exhibited in the right lower quadrant (RLQ) of the abdomen below the belly button (or movement of pain from mid to right side). McBurney's point refers to the point of maximum tenderness in the RLQ that is a sign of acute appendicitis. While Psoas sign is the irritation of the iliopsoas muscles in the hip flexor that is a sign of retrocecal appendicitis (ie. the appendix doesn't protrude out but is instead within the large intestine).

Causes of Metabolic Acidosis

LUSK

L — **Lactic**

buildup of lactic acid producued by muscle/RBCs

U — **Uremic**

kidney disease; failure to filter out acid from blood

S — **Salicylate**

salicylate poisoning eg. via aspirin overdose

K — **Ketoacidosis**

excessive conversion of fat to (acidic) ketone bodies

Tip: Recall the ROME mnemonic used to interpret ABG results whereby a sign of metabolic acidosis is that pH and HCO3 are both low or both high.

Signs of Portal Hypertension

ABCDE

A	Ascites
B	Bleeding
C	Caput medusa
D	Decreased albumin
E	Enlarged spleen

Symptoms of Dumping Syndrome

DAT

D	Dizziness
A	Abdominal cramping
T	Tachycardia

Causes of (Anion Gap) Metabolic Acidosis

GOLDMARK

G	Glycols (Specifically ethylene glycol and propylene glycol)
O	Oxoproline
L	L-lactate
D	D-lactate
M	Methanol
A	Aspirin
R	Renal failure or uremia
K	Ketoacidosis

This will help you remember the causes of anion gap metabolic acidosis, which is when kidneys are not removing enough acid from the body.

Risk Factors of Cholelithiasis

FFFFF

F	Fat
F	Forty
F	Fertile
F	Female
F	Fair

The five F's as a mnemonic device are designed to help nurses and nursing students understand the risk factors of cholelithiasis, or gallstones. Cholelithiasis has several risk factors, but these are frankly the most common. The commonly cited causes are higher estrogen levels (and oral contraceptive use) in women; the high significance of cholesterol in the formation of gallstones; and high calorie, high glycemic load, "western" diets.

Topics: Oncology

Key Indicators of Cancer

CAUTION UP

C — **Change**
Specifically change in bowel movements or the bladder.

A — **A lesion**
A tear or cut that will not heal.

U — **Unusual bleeding**
Specifically vaginal bleeding or other types of discharge.

T — **Thickening**
Generally a thickness of the skin or a lump that can be detected in tissue, such as the breast.

I — **Indigestion**
Regular upset stomach or difficulty swallowing.

O — **Obvious**
Changes in skin, such as in a new or growing wart or mole.

N — **Nagging coughs**
Watch for a hoarseness that will not go away.

U — **Unexplained weight loss**
Loss of appetite can also be an indicator.

P — **Pernicious anemia**
Check for a deficiency of B12 in the blood.

Leukemia Symptoms

ANT

A	Anemia
N	Neutropenia
T	Thrombocytopenia

Cheat Sheet

Topics in Medicine

Cheat Sheet

Topics in Medicine

Labs & Interpretation

Basic Metabolic Panel Normal Labs

Sodium	Odd numbers = 1, 3, 5 = 135	135-145 mEq/L
Potassium	3-5 bananas/bunch	3.5-5 mEq/L
BUN	BUNion: 5 toes/fingers, 20 total	5-20 mg/dL
Creatinine	creatinNINE (0.9 is middle)	0.6-1.2 mg/dL
Glucose	Energy lower at 70-100yrs old	70-100
Calcium	Gallon of milk weighs 8.5lbs (+2)	8.5-10.5 mg/dL
Chloride	Hot tub temperatures (F)	95-105 mEq/L
Bicarbonate	Buying 12-pack of soda x 2 = 24	23-29 mEq/L

Tip: Recall that the NCLEX assumes standard environmental conditions such as being at sea level (altitude can heavily affect creatinine, bicarbonates... among other markers.) Even having a rough intuition about the normal range for all labs is helpful as NCLEX questions typically present lab values that deviate very noticeably from the normal range.

Complete Blood Count Normal Labs

WBC	Wanna Buy a (old) Car: $5k-10k	5,000-10,000/mcL
RBC	Adult human body has ~4.5-5.5L	4.5-5.5mill./mcL
Hemoglobin	Hemoglobin carries oxygen. At rest, average adult takes 12-18 breaths/min	12-18 g/dL
Hematocrit	Mid life crisis years: 37-50	37-50%
Platelet	Gold plated sports car: $150-400k	150,000-400,000/mcL

Coagulation Study Normal Labs

INR	INR = 1NR → <1	<1
PT	PTen = 10	10-12 sec
PTT	PTenTwenty = 10+20 = 30	30-40 sec

Arterial Blood Gas Normal Labs

HCO3	Just graduated college ages	22-26 mEq/L
PaCO2	Midlife crisis ages	35-45 mmHg
Blood pH	PACO2: 35-45 / 100 = .35-.45 → 7.35-7.45	7.35-7.45
SaO2	straight As in school	95-100
PaO2	straight B-minuses in school	80-100

ABG Imbalance

ROME

R	Respiratory
O	Opposite Either the pH is low and the (acidic) pCO_2 is high or the pH is high and the pCO_2 is low
M	Metabolic
E	Equal Either both the pH and the (basic) HCO_3 will be low or the pH and the HCO_3 will be high.

"ROME" can be used to analyze arterial blood gas (ABG) results to identify the cause of an acid-base imbalance:

Respiratory: When the pH and PaCO2 values are opposite, indicating a respiratory disturbance

Metabolic: When the pH and HCO3 values are equal, indicating a metabolic disturbance

Common Abnormal Lab Values

PP in the COP 6 times for $40k

P	pH in 6's
P	Potassium in 6's
C	$CO_2 > 60$
O	$O_2 < 60$
P	Platelets < 40k

This mnemonic helps identify abnormal lab values via the number 6. To help remember, recall that pH and potassium levels are commonly measured in a urine (PP) sample, whereas platelet count can only be measured by a blood sample.

Other Normal Lab Values

P

Potassium:

3.5-5 (baby banana...)

C

Chloride:

95-105 (Hot tub temperatures, in F)

H

Hemoglobin Male:

13-18 (male puberty)

H

Hemoglobin Female:

12-16 (girls puberty, they go through first)

M

Magnesium:

1.5-2.5 (Magnet has 2 poles, halfway out each side +or- 0.5)

C

Calcium:

9-11: (911 whats your emergency? I need MILK!)

P

Phosphate:

2.5-4.5: These Phos-sils are 2.5-4.5 million years old!

Toxic Therapeudic Drug Levels

Rule of 2's

D Digitalis (digoxin): .5-2.5 = 2 range

L Lithium - .6-1.2 = 2x

T Theophylline - 10-20 = 2x

D Dilantin (Phenytoin)- 10-20 = 2x

Over these levels are TOXIC.

Lab Values indicating Neutropenia

WBCN

W	WBC: <1000
N	Neutrophils: <500

Tip: Recall that neutropenia thereby invokes neutropenic precautions mnemonic described in "Safety and Infection Control" to prevent infection in the immunocompromised client.

Lab Values for Statin Administration

CTLDLHDL

C Cholesterol <200

T Triglycerides <150

L LDLs <100

H HDLs > 60

ECG Presentation and Risks Reference

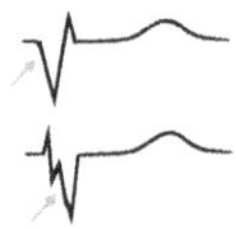

Q-Waves or fragmented QRS complexes

Evidence of previous myocardial infraction and high risk of ventricular tachcyardia and ventricular fibrillation.

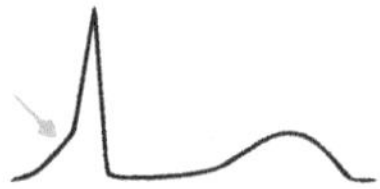

Delta wave, pre-excitation

Risk of AVRT. May be accompanied by atrial fibrillation (pre-excited atrial fibrillation).

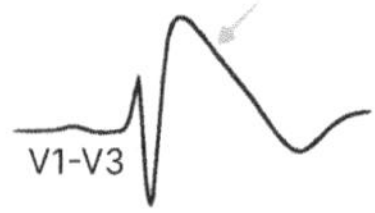

Brugada syndrome: ST elevation V1-V4. Shark tail appearance or saddle formed

Risk of ventricular tachycardia and ventricular fibrillation

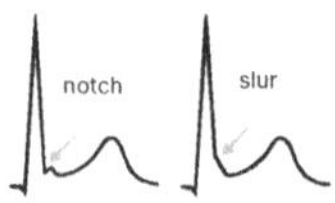

Early repolarization: slurring or notching at end-QRS

5 times increased risk of ventricular tachycardia and ventricular fibrillation.

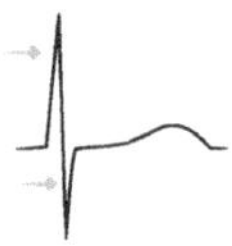

Hypertrophic cardiomyopathy: deep S, large R

Risk of ventricular tachycardia and ventricular fibrillation

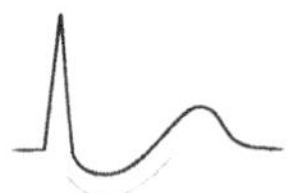

Digoxin effect: ST depression with "sagging" appearance

Digoxin may cause virtually all known arrhythmias

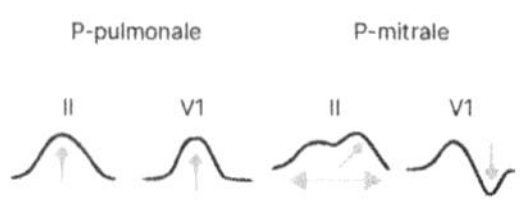

P- pulmonale (right atrial abnormality) and

P- mitrale (left atrial abnormality)

Associated with atrial tachyarrhythmias

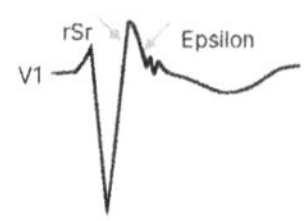

Arrhythmogenic right ventricular cardiomyopathy : rSr-pattern in V1 with epsilon wave after QRS

Risk of ventricular tachycardia and ventricular fibrillation

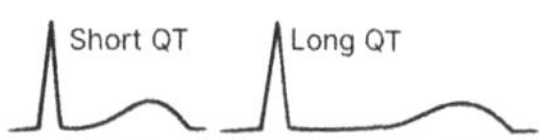

Long QT interval (LQTS) or Short QT interval (SQTS)

Long QT syndrome is fairly common and poses risk of ploymorphic ventricular tachycardia referred to as torsade de points. Short QT syndrome is very rare but may also cause torsade de pointes.

ECG Risks: Key Points

PQLSCB

P	Patrial (top floor)
Q	QRS = ventricular (bottom floor)
L	Lack of QRS asystole
S	Sawtooth appearance atrial flutter
C	Chaotic fibrillation
B	Bizarre tachycardia

6 L's of Possible Hypokalemia

6 L's

L	Lethargy
L	Leg cramps
L	Limp muscles
L	Low or shallow breathing
L	Lethal cardiac dysrhythmia
L	Lots of urine

Tip: Recall in cases of severe hypokalemia, if client isn't adequately urinating (30-60ml/hr), potassium can not be administered because it can cause renal damage. If client is urinating it can be IV infused slowly (≤20 mEq/hr) with oral administration preferred.

Causes and Signs of Hyperkalemia

MACHINE MURDER

M	Medication (ACE, NSAIDS)
A	Acidosis
C	Cellular destruction (burns)
H	Hypoaldosteronism
I	Intake of supplements
N	Nephron failure
E	Excretion impaired
M	Muscle weakness
U	Urinary changes (oliguria)
R	Respiratory distress
D	Decreased cardiac motility
E	EKG changes
R	Reflexes

Signs of Hypernatremia

FRIED

F	Fever (low-grade), flushed skin
R	Restless (irritable)
I	Increased fluid retention and increased BP
E	Edema (peripheral and pitting)
D	Decreased urinary output, dry mouth

Signs of Hypernatremia

SALT

S	Skin flushed
A	Agitation
L	Low-grade fever
T	Thirst

Signs of Hyponatremia

SALT LOSS

S	Stupor/coma
A	Anorexia, N/V
L	Lethargy
T	Tendon reflexes decreased
L	Limp muscles (weakness)
O	Orthostatic hypotension
S	Seizures/headache
S	Stomach cramping

Signs of Hypercalcemia

BSMGN

B	Bones demineralization,
S	Stones nephrolithiasis
M	Moans pain
G	Groans constipation
N	Neurons psychiatric symptoms

Signs of Hypocalcemia

CATS

C	Convulsions or Chvostek's sign
A	Arrhythmias
T	Tetany or Trosseau's sign
S	Spasms and stridor

Cheat Sheet

Labs & Interpretation

Pharmacology

Drug Antidotes

Warfarin K	**Warfarin:** Vitamin K
Acetacysteine	**Acetaminophen:** Acetylcysteine
Opioxone	**Opioids:** Naloxone
Aspirin Bicarb	**Aspirin:** Sodium bicarbonate
Magnesium Gluco	**Magnesium sulfate:** Calcium gluconate
Hepasulfate	**Heparin:** Protamine sulfate

Common Emergency Drugs

"drugs to LEAN on"

L	**Lidocaine** Injections of this drug can help to treat ventricular arrhythmias.
E	**Epinephrine** Injected to assist with cardiac or respiratory emergencies, such as anaphylaxis.
A	**Atropine sulfate** Injections of this drug are used to treat sinus bradycardia or reverse the effects of certain anticholinesterase medications.
N	**Narcan** Injected to treat opioid overdoses.

Signs of Lidocaine Toxicity

SAMS

S	Slurred speech
A	Altered central nervous system
M	Muscle twitching
S	Seizures

Despite being generally safe for use as a topical anesthetic, lidocaine can be harmful if used incorrectly or excessively. This can occur in clinical environments such as in operating rooms. The systemic toxicity is typically treated by emergency administration of lipid emulsion therapy to sequester lidocaine (a lipophilic medication,) and benzodiazepines

Common Negative Symptoms of Birth Control

SEA CASH

S	Severe leg pain
E	Eye issues
A	Abdominal pain
C	Chest pain
A	Acne
S	Swelling of ankles and feet
H	Headaches

Rhythm Disorder Treatments

ABCD's

A	Adenosine
B	Beta Blockers
C	Calcium Channel Blockers
D	Digoxin

Drugs to Treat Bradycardia/ Hypotension

IDEA

I	Isoproterenol
D	Dopamine
E	Epinephrine
A	Atropine Sulfate

Symptoms Treated by Thiazides

CHIC

C	Congestive Heart Failure
H	Hypertension
I	Insipidus
C	Calcium calculi

Thiazides are the most commonly used oral diuretic often first recommended for the treatment of high blood pressure (hypertension), or to clear excess fluid from the body (edema) in the case of congestive heart failure. Common thiazide diuretics are chlorothiazide and hydrochlorothiazide though thiazide-like diuretics like metolazone, indapamide, and chlorthalidone.

Side Effects of Morphine

MORPHINE

M	Myosis
O	Out of it (sedated)
R	Respiratory depression
P	Pneumonia
H	Hypotension
I	Infrequency
N	Nausea
E	Emesis vomiting

Drugs Treating Ventricular Arrythmias

PALS

P	Procainamide
A	Amiodarone
L	Lidocaine
S	Sotalol

Treatment of Myocardial Infraction

MONA BAH

M — **Morphine**
For pain relief and anxiety reduction.

O — **Oxygen**
If the patient is hypoxic.

N — **Nitroglycerin**
To relieve chest pain and improve blood flow.

A — **Aspirin**
To prevent further clotting.

B — **Beta-Blockers**
To reduce heart rate, blood pressure, and myocardial oxygen demand.

A — **ACE Inhibitors/ARBs**
To reduce blood pressure and decrease the heart's workload.

H — **Heparin**
An anticoagulant to prevent new clots from forming

Drugs Treating HIV

ZZ-LSD

Z	Zidovudine
Z	Zalcitabine
L	Lamivudine
S	Stavudine
D	Didanosine

Treatment of Congestive Heart Failure

MADD DOG

M	Morphine
A	Aminophylline
D	Digoxin
D	Dopamine
D	Diuretics
O	Oxygen
G	Gasses (gasses is for monitoring the arterial blood gasses)

Tip: A common presentation of CHF is via pulmonary edema (accumulation of fluid in the air sacs of the lungs, making it difficult to breathe), since inefficient pumping in CHF increases pressure in lung veins, pushing fluid into lung's air sacs.

6 S's of Steroid Side Effects

6 S's

S — **Sugar**
hyperglycemia

S — **Soggy bones**
osteoporosis

S — **Sic**
decreased immunity

S — **Sad**
depression

S — **Salt**
water and salt retention (hypertension)

S — **Sex**
decreased libido

Common Parkinson's Medications

Ali Loves Boxing MAO-tches

A	Amantadine
L	Levodopa
B	Bromocriptine
M	MAO inhibitors

Asthma Common Treatments

ASTHMA

A	Adrenergic (albuterol)
S	Steroids
T	Theophylline
H	Hydration (IV)
M	Mask (oxygen)
A	Antibiotics

Using Beta Blockers

B1 vs B2

This mnemonic is designed to help nursing students remember which beta-blockers to use. B1 is for the heart (B-ecause we have 1 heart) and B2 is for the lungs (B-ecause we have 2 lungs).

Beta Blocker Contraindications

ABCDE

A	Asthma
B	Block (heart block)
C	COPD
D	Diabetes mellitus
E	Electrolyte (hyperkalemia)

Bradycardia Treatment

IDEA

I	Isoproterenol
D	Dopamine
E	Epinephrine
A	Atropine sulfate

Common Drugs that Interact

These Drugs Can Interact

T	Theophylline
D	Dilantin
C	Coumadin
I	Ilosone

Anti-TB drugs

RIPES

R	Rifampicin
I	Isoniazid
P	Pyrazinamide
E	Ethambutol
S	Streptomycin

Warfarin Drug Interactions

ACADEMIC QACS

A	Amiodarone
C	Cimetidine
A	Aspirin
D	Dapsone
E	Erythromycin
M	Metronidazole
I	Indomethacin
C	Clofibrates
Q	Quinidine
A	Azapropazone
C	Ciprofloxacin
S	Statins

ACE Inhibitor Side Effects

TROPICAL P

T — Taste
diminished or distorted sense of taste

R — Renal insufficiency
(kidney problems)

O — Orthostatic ↓BP
(hypotension→tired, dizzy)

P — Potassium (↑K+)
hyperkalemia

I — Impotence

C — (dry) Cough

A — Anaphylaxis

L — Leucocytosis
high white blood cell count

P — Palpitations

Treatment For Hypertension

ABCDE

A	Ace inihibitors/ARBs
B	Beta blockers
C	Calcium blockers
D	Diuretics
E	Electrolyte (hyperkalemia)

Early Signs Of Digoxin Toxicity

BAD VAN

B	Bradycardia/Tachycardia
A	Anorexia
D	Diarrhea
V	Visual disturbances
A	Abdominal Cramps
N	Nausea and vomiting

5 S's of Corticosteroid Side Effects

5 S's

S	**Sick** easier to get sick
S	**Sad** causes depression
S	**Sex** increases libido
S	**Salt** retains more and causes weight gain
S	**Sugar** raises blood sugar

Comprehensive Side Effects Of Steroids

My BABy DASCHUNDS

M	Moon face (face swells, gets rounder)
B	Bone loss
A	Appetite (increase)
B	Buffalo Hump
D	Depression
A	Acne
S	Striae (stretch marks)
C	Cataracts
H	Hypertension
U	Up all night
N	Necrosis (avascular)
D	DM
S	Suppression of adrenal

3 S's of Sulfonamide Side Effects

3 S's

S Steven Johnson syndrome
painful/spreading rash, blisters, emergency

S Skin rash

S Shiny crystals in urine

Drugs Causing Agranulocytosis

3 C's

C	Clozapine
C	Colchicine
C	Carbamazepine

Parkinson's Treatment Drugs

SALA

S Seligiline
(Eldepryl)

A Anticholinergics
(Cogentin, Artane)

L L-Dopa
(Sinemet)

A Amantadine
(Symmetryl)

Drugs for Seizures

C++ ("C"-plus -plus)

C	Carbamazepine
P	Phenytoin
P	Phenobarbital

Drugs Causing Cataracts

ABCD

A	Amiodarone
B	Busulfan
C	Chlorpromazine
D	Dexamethasone

Osmotic Diuretics

GUM

G	Glycerol
U	Urea
M	Mannitol

Psychiatric Meds Common Side Effects

"A-B-C-D-E-F-G, psy-chi-a-tric-me-di-cine"

A Anticholinergic effects (dry mouth)

B Blurred vision

C Constipation

D Drowsiness

E Euphoria

F F/Ph-otophobia

G Granulocytosis (lower WBC)

Lithium Toxicity Symptoms

"lithium metal diarrhea earthquake"

Metal	Metallic: metallic taste
Diarrhea	Diarrhea: diarrhea
Earthquake	Earthquake: tremors

Anticoagulant Administration Criteria

Warfarin	Heparin
• Maintenance oral anticoagulant. Measure PT/INR. • PT/INR: 0.8-1.1	• Anticoagulant given through IV or SQ. Measure aPTT levels. • aPTT level: 30-40 normally, or 60-80 seconds on heparin.

Antibiotics Contraindications During Pregnancy

MCAT

M	Metronidazole
C	Chloramphenicol
A	Aminoglycoside
T	Tetracycline

Drugs That Can Cause Hyperkalemia

K BANK

K	K-sparing diuretics
B	Beta blockers
A	ACE inhibitors
N	NSAIDs
K	K-supplements

Hyperkalemia Treatment

KIND

K	Kayexalate via oral or enema
I	Insulin
N	$NaHCO_3$
D	Diuretics Furosemide & Thiazides

Common Drugs Inducing SLE (Lupus) Symptoms

Quinn the HIP MD

Q Quinidine (antiarrhythmic)

H Hydralazine (treats high BP)

I Isoniazi (antibiotic, treats TB)

P Procainamide (antiarrhythmic)

M Minocycline (antibiotic)

D Diltiazem (treats high BP)

Drugs Causing QT Prolongation

APACHE

A	Amiodarone (antiarrythmic)
P	Procainamide (antiarrythmic)
A	Arsenic Trioxide (leukemia)
C	Cisapride (GI movement)
H	Haloperidol (antipsychotic)
E	Erythromycin (antibiotic)

Drugs Causing Gynecomastia

DISCOS

D	Digoxin
I	Isoniazid
S	Spironolocatone
C	Cimetidine
O	Oestrogens
S	Stillbestrol

Thrombolytic Agents

USA

U	Urokinase
S	Streptokinase
A	Alteplase (t-PA)

Cheat Sheet

Pharmacology

Make-Your-Own-Mnemonic

Make-Your-Own-Mnemonic

Make-Your-Own-Mnemonic

Make-Your-Own-Mnemonic

Make-Your-Own-Mnemonic

Made in United States
Orlando, FL
20 August 2026

86216561R00134